Low Carb

*Ultimate Healthy Low Carb Diet Recipes
to reclaim your health*

(Healthy Cooking with Low Carb Diet meal plans)

Cecil Jennings

Published by Jason Thawne Publishing House

© Cecil Jennings

Low Carb: Ultimate Healthy Low Carb
Diet Recipes to reclaim your health (Healthy
Cooking with Low Carb Diet meal plans)

All Rights Reserved

ISBN 978-1-989749-24-1

This document is geared towards providing exact and reliable information in regards to the topic and issue covered. The publication is sold with the idea that the publisher isn't required to render accounting, officially permitted, or otherwise, qualified services. If advice is necessary, legal or even professional, a practiced individual in the profession should be ordered.

- From a Declaration of Principles which was accepted and approved equally by a Committee of the American Bar Association and a Committee of Publishers and Associations.

In no way is it legal to reproduce, duplicate, or even transmit any part of this document in either electronic means or in printed format. Recording of this publication is strictly prohibited and any storage of this document isn't allowed unless with proper written permission from the publisher. All rights reserved.

The information provided herein is stated to be truthful and consistent, in that any liability, in terms of inattention or otherwise, by any usage or abuse of any policies, processes, or directions contained within is the solitary and also utter responsibility of the recipient reader. Under no circumstances will any legal responsibility or blame be held against the publisher for any reparation, damages, or monetary loss due to the information herein, either directly or indirectly.

Respective authors own all copyrights not held by the publisher.

The information herein is offered for just informational purposes solely, and is universal as so. The presentation of the information is without contract or any type of guarantee assurance.

The trademarks that are used are without any consent, and also the publication of the trademark is without permission or backing by the trademark owner. All trademarks and brands within this book are for clarifying purposes only and are the owned by the owners themselves, not affiliated with this document.

TABLE OF CONTENTS

Part 1 1

Spicy India Omelet 2

Spectacular Spinach Omelet 2

Outstanding Veggie Omelet 2

Spicy Spinach Bake..2

Delish Veggie Hash With Eggs..3

Eggs, Mushrooms And Onion Bonanza....................................4

Zucchini Casserole 5

Low Carb Pumpkin Spice Pancakes 6

Apple Buckwheat Muffins 7

Low Carb Banana Strawberry Breakfast Cookies 8

Low Carb Grain Free Baked Porridge 9

Low Carb Breakfast Stir Fry Recipe 10

Low Carb Pumpkin Pancakes..11

Eggplant With Eggs 12

Spicy Granola..13

Divine Protein Muesli...14

Healthy Bean Soup...15

Un-Fried Crispy Baked Beet Chips..16

Easy Low Fat Cheddar 17

- Crisp Baked Radish Chips 18
- Eggplant Jerky Snack 18
- Homemade Baked Cinnamon-Flavored Apple Chips 20
- Breakfast Burritos 20
- Scrambled Eggs 22
- Sausage Gravy 23
- Ultimate Granola 23
- Tasty Apple Almond Coconut Medley 24
- Scrambled Eggs With Chili 25
- Basil And Walnut Eggs Divine 26
- Spicy Scrambled Eggs 26
- Spicy India Omelet 27
- Spectacular Spinach Omelet 28
- Part 2 30
- Introduction 31
- Chapter 1: Before Anything Else 32
- Chapter 2: Getting Started 44
- Your New Plate 46
- Chapter 3: Low Carb Style Food Shopping 56
- Conclusion 71
- About The Author 73

Part 1

Spicy India Omelet
Spectacular Spinach Omelet
Outstanding Veggie Omelet

Ingredients
- 3 scallions, sliced diagonal
- 3 eggs, beaten
- Salt to taste
- 1 handful tiny broccoli
- 1 carrot, matchstick cut
- **Safflower oil**

Directions
- Raise the temperature of oil in a skillet.
- Add the sliced carrots and broccoli florets in the warm oil and stir it.
- Gently add eggs and scallions and keeping on stirring it with a spatula.
- *Add a pinch of salt and pepper to enhance taste.*

Spicy Spinach Bake

Ingredients
- 1 bunch fresh spinach, shopped
- Hot pepper flakes (½ tsp)
- 6 eggs

- Olive oil
- **Pepper and salt to taste**

Directions
- Heat the olive oil in a skillet on a stove.
- Put hot pepper flakes.
- In a separate bowl, beat the eggs and combine pepper, spinach and salt.
- Transfer the mixture to the hot pepper flakes and cook.
- Occasionally flip the mixture to cook it from both the sides.
- *Let it cool for some time and garnish with coriander leaves!*

Delish Veggie Hash With Eggs

Ingredients
- Sweet white onion (¼ cup), chopped
- Pepper and salt to taste
- 2 cloves garlic, minced
- Fresh spinach (1 cup), chopped
- Cherry tomatoes (1 cup), halved
- Mushroom (½ cup), sliced
- Extra virgin olive oil (2 tablespoon)
- 4 eggs, cooked
- **Yellow squash (1 cup), chopped**

Directions
- Heat olive oil in a skillet and sauté onion and garlic for about 2 minutes.
- Add chopped squash and cook for 2 more minutes.
- Add mushrooms to the mixture and cook for another five minutes.
- Flavor it with pepper and salt.
- Then add spinach and tomatoes until spinach wilts and then drain.
- *Serve along with cooked eggs and enjoy!*

Eggs, Mushrooms And Onion Bonanza

Ingredients
- 12 hard boiled eggs, peeled and finely chopped
- Ground black pepper to taste
- 12 medium white mushrooms, finely chopped
- 1 medium onion, finely diced
- **Coconut oil (¼ cup)**

Directions

- Kick start the recipe by heating coconut oil in a pan; sauté onions till it transforms its color to brown.
- Add mushrooms and sauté for 5 more minutes and stir continuously.
- Turn off the flame and let it cool.
- Finally add eggs to the mixture and sprinkle some pepper.
- *Enjoy the mouth watering bonanza!*

Zucchini Casserole

Ingredients
- 5 eggs
- 3 large zucchini
- Mushrooms (½ cup)
- ½ red onion, chopped
- **Pepper and salt to taste**

Directions
- Take a bowl and blend the eggs with a beater along with salt and pepper.
- In another bowl, finely grate the zucchini.

- Jumble both the mixtures into each other.
- Heat olive oil in a pan and pour the above mixture in it.
- Cover the pan with its lid and let it cook for 5 minutes.
- Bake it for about 15 minutes in the preheated oven at 375 degrees Fahrenheit.
- *Cool for some time and then serve!*

Low Carb Pumpkin Spice Pancakes

Ingredients
- Cinnamon powder (1 tbsp)
- Honey
- Water (½ cup + 3 tbsp)
- Uncooked oatmeal (½ cup)
- Cinnamon powder (1 tbsp)
- 2 egg whites
- Baking powder (½ tbsp)
- Shredded pumpkin (½ cup), cooked
- **Protein powder (1 scoop)**

Direction

- In a serving bowl, intermingle all the dry ingredients and sift them first.
- Take a blender and mix all the dry and wet ingredients until it forms a smooth paste.
- Pour cooking oil in a pan and empty the batter into it.
- Cook until it turns golden brown.
- *Relish the food with honey!*

Apple Buckwheat Muffins

Ingredients
- Baking powder (1 tbsp)
- Buckwheat flour (¼ cup)
- Salt (1/8 tsp), course
- Cinnamon powder (½ tbsp)
- Walnuts (¼ cup), chopped
- ½ piece banana, mashed
- 2 eggs (large and farm fresh)
- Honey (¼ cup)
- **½ Sweet apple, finely diced**

Direction
- Preheat the oven to 350 F.

- Whisk cinnamon, baking powder, salt and flour together in a large bowl and mix well.
- In another bowl, mix the wet ingredients like honey, banana and egg until it turns to a creamy smooth mixture.
- Combine both dry and wet ingredients before folding in apples and walnuts.
- Meanwhile, prepare the baking cups in a muffin tin and then fill the batter in the cups.
- Bake for about 30 minutes in the preheated oven until the toothpick comes out clean.
- *Serve and relish the appetite!*

Low Carb Banana Strawberry Breakfast Cookies

Ingredients
- Sea salt (¼ tsp)
- Almond butter (½ cup)
- Coconut flour (¼ cup)
- Cinnamon (½ tsp)
- Chopped raisins (2 tbsp)
- Chopped pecans (2 tbsp)

- Diced strawberry (2 tbsp)
- 6 whole dates soaked and pitted in hot water
- 2 medium eggs lightly beaten
- Nutmeg (1 tsp)
- 2 bananas, mashed
- Unsweetened shredded coconut (½ cup)
- **Baking powder (½ tsp)**

Directions

- Take a food processor and process coconut, almond butter and dates.
- Now add baking powder, eggs, salt, cinnamon and shredded coconut and keep on beating for 30 seconds.
- Softly fold in raisins, strawberries and pecans once shifted to a bowl.
- Take the parchment paper lining with a cookie sheet and scoop the dough by tablespoon on it.
- *Press each cookie and bake for about 15 minutes at 350 degrees Fahrenheit until golden brown.*

Low Carb Grain Free Baked Porridge

Ingredients
- Unsweetened coconut (1 cup)
- 2 eggs
- Raw honey (¼ cup)
- Milk (1 ½ cups)
- Crushed pecans (1 cup)
- Cinnamon (1 ½ tsp)
- **Sea salt (1 tsp)**

Directions
- Separately mix the wet ingredients and the dry ones.
- Bring both together and blend well.
- Take casserole dish, shift the mixture to it and bake in the preheated oven at 350 degrees Fahrenheit for about 25-30 minutes.
- Add milk and garnish it with honey to enhance the taste.
- *Serve chilled!*

Low Carb Breakfast Stir Fry Recipe

Ingredients
- Minced garlic (1 tsp)
- Coconut oil (1 tsp)
- 4 eggs

- Spinach (4 cups)
- Leeks (1 cup), chopped
- **Chopped carrot (½ cup)**

Directions
- Heat oil in a frying pan on the stove.
- Beat the eggs in a bowl and season it with salt and pepper.
- Pour the mixture on the heated oil like an omelet and serve when completely cooked from both sides.
- Take a separate frying pan to cook carrot, garlic and leeks in it.
- Add spinach and cook it further.
- Gently spread the mixture over the already cooked omelet.
- *Serve hot with green chilies to spice it up!*

Low Carb Pumpkin Pancakes

Ingredients
- Pure maple syrup (¼ cup)
- Flax seed (½ cup)
- Coconut oil (2 tbsp)

- 4 eggs
- Pumpkin puree (1 cup)
- Almond flour (2 cups)
- Cinnamon (1 tsp)
- Vinegar (1 tsp)
- Almond milk (½ cup)
- Sea salt (½ tsp)
- Baking soda (½ tsp)
- **Pumpkin pie spice (1 tsp)**

Directions

- Heat coconut oil in a skillet preferably a non stick one.
- Merge the dry ingredients separately and the wet ingredients separately in another bowl.
- Combine both gradually and stir smoothly to avoid lumps.
- Drop one large spoonful into the pan and fry on each side until golden brown.
- *Serve with maple syrup either hot or chilled!*

Eggplant With Eggs

Ingredients

- 3 medium eggs
- 2 eggplants, sliced into discs
- Pepper and salt to taste
- **Coconut oil for frying**

Directions

- Heat the coconut oil in a skillet.
- Beat the eggs smooth with a beater and dip each disc of egg plant in it.
- Take out the disc, put into the frying pan and fry until golden brown.
- *Serve hot with sour cream or sauce!*

Spicy Granola

Ingredients

- Hemp seeds (¼ cups)
- Cinnamon (2 tsp)
- Almond flour (1 ½ cups)
- Coconut flakes (½ cup)
- Walnuts (½ cup)
- Coconut oil (1/3 cup)
- Salt to taste
- **Nutmeg (2 tsp)**

Directions

- Preheat the oven to 275 degrees Fahrenheit.
- Mix all the ingredients in a large bowl and then spread on a greased baking sheet.
- Bake for about 40 minutes and then allow cooling for sometime before serving.
- *Spicy Granola is ready!*

Divine Protein Muesli

Ingredients

- Chocolate chips (1 tbsp)
- Hemp protein (1 tbsp)
- Unsweetened almond milk (1 cup)
- Chopped walnuts (1 tbsp)
- Coconut flakes (1 cup), unsweetened
- Cinnamon (½ tsp)
- **Raw almonds (1 tbsp)**

Directions

- It is again a very simple yet rich in taste recipe.
- Take a bowl and layer coconut flakes, chocolate chips, raisins, walnuts and almonds.

- Sprinkle cinnamon powder; an ingredient that helps in weight loss. Pour milk over it.
- *Serve with crushed almonds at the top!*

Healthy Bean Soup

Ingredients
- Chicken broth (4 cups)
- Italian herb seasoning (2 tsp)
- Shredded Cheddar cheese
- Chopped parsley (1 cup)
- Navy beans (2 cans of 15 ounces), undrained, split
- Raw kale (4 cups), chopped
- Pepper and salt according to taste
- 1 medium yellow onion, chopped
- 8 garlic cloves, minced
- Olive oil (1 tbsp)
- Diced tomatoes (1 can)
- **Sliced carrots (2 cans), undrained**

Direction
- Heat olive oil in a pan and sauté onion and garlic in it until tender.
- Add kale and cook further for 15 minutes until wilted.

- Add pepper, salt, tomatoes, carrots, beans, broth (3 cups) and herbs and let it simmer for 5 minutes.
- Blend the veggies in a blender and then simmer for 15 minutes more.
- Shift the mixture to the bowl, splash with chopped parsley and Cheddar cheese and serve with crust bread.
- *The healthy low carb soup is done!*

Un-Fried Crispy Baked Beet Chips

Ingredients
- Non-stick cooking spray
- 4 large beets, scrubbed clean
- **Salt according to taste**

Directions
- Before initiating, preheat the oven to 375F.
- Cut the beet, molding them to potato chips.
- Take the cookie sheet spray; evenly place the sliced beets on it.
- Flavor it with salt or any other seasoning.

- The mixture is ready to be roasted. Place it in the oven for 45-60 minutes.
- It can be served with any sour cream or the favorite dip of your choice.
- *Eat and relish!*

Easy Low Fat Cheddar

Ingredients
- Becel topping and cooking spray
- Zucchini (1 cup), sliced
- **Cheddar cheese (1 tbsp), grated**

Direction
- Take a cookie sheet and spray evenly with cooking spray.
- Take the other ingredients; Becel, Cheddar cheese and Zucchini and put them in a sealed foil or bag.
- Shake them all so well that they get over each other.
- Cook the mixture till the cheese melts and it turns to brownish color.

- *Take it out in a platter and serve hot for a better taste.*

Crisp Baked Radish Chips

Ingredients
- Non-stick cooking spray
- Pepper and salt to taste
- **10-15 large radishes**

Directions
- Preheat the oven to 375 F.
- Take cookie sheet and splash with non-stick cooking spray.
- Cut the radishes to make fine thin chips and place them evenly on the cooking sheet.
- Sprinkle black pepper and salt.
- Bake both the sides one by one for 10 minutes.
- Take it out when it gets crispy and golden in color.
- Serve hot or let it cool down.
- *Splash lemon juice to taste even good.*

Eggplant Jerky Snack

Ingredients

- Maple syrup (2 tbsp)
- Olive oil (¾ cup)
- 1 ripe eggplant (about a pound), washed
- Vinegar (3 tbsp)
- Paprika (1 tsp)
- **Salt according to taste**

Direction

- Take the egg plant and cut it length wise. Then finely cut it further into thin strips.
- Take maple syrup, vinegar and oil and beat them well in a large bowl.
- Marinate the egg plant strips with this mixture.
- Leave it for two hours so that the egg plant completely takes in the coating.
- Take a baking sheet and arrange the cut strips on it. Sprinkle salt over it.
- Bake it for 10-12 minutes. Keep on turning its sides to avoid burning.
- After it is done completely, place it in a zip lock bag to absorb extra oil.
- *The delicious jerky snack is ready to be enjoyed.*

Homemade Baked Cinnamon-Flavored Apple Chips

Ingredients
- 2 apples
- **Cinnamon (2 tbsp)**

Direction
- Preheat the oven to 200 degrees Celsius.
- Take the apple, peel it off and remove seeds.
- Thinly slice the apple to fine strips.
- Arrange the apple slices on a baking sheet.
- Splash some cinnamon, a magic ingredient that aids in weight loss.
- Bake it for an hour on each side.
- *Enjoy the low carb recipe to fill your appetite!*

Breakfast Burritos

Ingredients
- Beef sausage (1 lb), cooked
- 24 wheat tortillas
- Cheddar cheese (2 cups), shredded

- Chunky salsa (½ cup)
- **12 beaten eggs**

Optional Ingredients

- 2 green onions
- 1 tomato, peeled and chopped
- 1 onion, finely diced
- 1-2 garlic clove, finely minced
- Chopped green chilies (4 ounce)
- Sliced jalapeno
- 6 potatoes, shredded and fried
- **1 green pepper, finely diced**

Direction

- Warm the Tortillas in the microwave oven for 20-30 seconds.
- Take all the sausages, salsa and eggs. Beat them altogether in a bowl.
- Gently pour ½ cup of the beaten eggs combination in the Tortillas rolling them in burrito form.
- Take a cookie sheet, grease it with a cooking brush and wrap up the burrito in it.
- Refrigerate it for some time.
- Use the optional ingredients to spice it up according to your taste.

- Bake it for almost 2 minutes before serving.
- *Cut into desired shape or serve as it is!*

Scrambled Eggs

Ingredients

- Water (1 tbsp)
- Sour cream (2 tbsp)
- Cheddar cheese (½ - ¾ cup), grated
- Butter (2 tbsp)
- Ground black pepper and salt according to taste
- **8 eggs**

Direction

- Take a serving bowl and beat the eggs well in it. Slowly add water and sour cream.
- Sprinkle a small amount of pepper and salt, beat lightly and put it aside.
- Take a frying pan and melt the butter on it, keeping the flame from low to medium.
- Gently add the egg mixture with constant stirring to avoid lumps.
- Finally add cheese and cook for another couple of minutes.

- *Serve when it comes to normal temperature. Enjoy!*

Sausage Gravy

Ingredients
- Milk (1 quart)
- Beef sausage (1 lb)
- Pillsbury Grands refrigerated buttermilk biscuits
- Pepper (1 dash)
- **Flour (1/3 cup)**

Direction
- Put the sausage in a frying pan and add some flour over it and cook for 5 minutes.
- Add milk and cook further to make it a thick fine paste.
- *Sprinkle some pepper ad serve with the buttermilk biscuits.*

Ultimate Granola

Ingredients
- Pecan pieces (1 tsp)
- Raw pumpkin seeds (1 tsp)
- Raw sunflower (1 tsp)

- Raw pine nuts (1 tsp)
- Coconut milk (1 cup)
- Fresh berries (2 tbsp)
- Slivered almonds (1 tsp)
- Walnut pieces (1 tsp)
- **Unsalted pistachios (1 tsp)**

Directions

- In a serving bowl, put the seeds and nuts in it first.
- *Now add milk and berries, mix it smooth and reserve it for some time until the mixture turns into the color released by berries.*

Tasty Apple Almond Coconut Medley

Ingredients

- Handful of unsweetened coconut
- One-half apple cored and roughly diced
- 1 pinch of salt
- Handful of sliced almonds
- **Generous dose of cinnamon**

Directions

- Take a blender and blend all the mentioned ingredients until it turns to a smoothie.
- *Serve cold with coconut milk!*

Scrambled Eggs With Chili

Ingredients
- 1 small onion, finely chopped and peeled
- Coconut milk (¼ cup)
- 6 eggs
- Coconut oil (2 tbsp)
- 4 fresh green chilies
- **Salt (¼ tsp)**

Directions
- Form the batter by blending eggs with salt and coconut milk. Set it aside.
- Take the green chilies and dispose off their seeds and peel their skin too.
- Heat oil in the skillet and cook the egg batter.
- Sprinkle the grated chilies over it.
- Stir it well until the eggs get cooked.

- *Serve the appetizing scrambled eggs hot!*

Basil And Walnut Eggs Divine

Ingredients
- Walnuts (1/3 cup), chopped
- Fresh basil (½ cup), chopped
- 3 eggs
- **Pepper and salt to taste**

Directions
- Cook eggs in a frying pan.
- Put together basil and cook further while stirring.
- To add taste, sprinkle salt and pepper.
- *Finley chop the walnuts and drizzle them over the mixture while serving.*

Spicy Scrambled Eggs

Ingredients
- 1 medium green pepper, cored, seeded and finely chopped
- 3 ripe tomatoes, peeled, seeded and chopped

- Ground black pepper and salt according to taste
- 1 red onion, finely chopped
- Extra virgin olive oil (1 tbsp)
- 4 large eggs
- **1 chile, seeded and cut into strips**

Directions

- Pre heat oil in a frying pan and cook onion until they turn brown.
- Prefer using a non stick skillet.
- Add chilies and pepper and cook with constant stirring.
- Now add tomatoes and use the seasonings of your choice; preferably salt and pepper.
- At the end, simply add eggs and cover the lid of the pan until everything gets cooked.
- *Serve hot!*

Spicy India Omelet

Ingredients

- 1 onion, chopped
- 3 eggs, beaten

- Coconut grated (¼ cup)
- 4 green chili
- **Oil for cooking**

Directions
- Pre heat the oil in a frying pan.
- Merge grated coconut with beaten eggs, salt, green chili and chopped onion.
- Pour the mixture in the pan in small amounts and cook the alternate sides.
- *Serve and add more chilies if required!*

Spectacular Spinach Omelet

Ingredients
- Tomato and onion salsa (1/3 cup)
- Cilantro (1 tbsp)
- 2 eggs, beaten
- Coconut oil (1 tbsp)
- **Raw spinach (1 ½ cups)**

Directions
- This light and yummy omelet is a perfect start for the day.
- Initialize by heating the coconut oil in the frying pan.

- Cook spinach until it loses water and gets soft.
- Put on the beaten eggs in the pan and cook until it gets mixed with the spinach.
- *Add salsa and splash with cilantro before serving.*

Part 2

Introduction

This isn't one of my typical topics that I deal with but I'm always getting asked if I've tried low carb dieting, whether it works and how easy is it really to do.

So rather than ignore all the fanfare about this much touted lifestyle, I thought I'd create this simple and "easy to swallow," guide to get people on the right track to losing weight quickly and easily with low carb.

Although initially it can be a bit of a hurdle to stop eating pizza, pasta and bread, you'll find that there are so many amazing and delicious foods that you can eat and still lose weight. This isn't called the starvation diet, it's low carbohydrate and it works.

The best part is that you've already started your journey to building a better you by downloading this book.

Chapter 1: Before Anything Else

Thinking about going low carb? Before you start on anything, it's important to know what you're getting yourself into. Going on a low-carb diet is easy and rewarding, but challenging. Going through it with head first, isn't going to do any good. Take these helpful tips to get you started.

BEFORE GOING ON A LOW-CARB DIET

Gather Valid Resources

You should be able to understand why you're making these food choices. Otherwise, how will you be able to inform others and rally their support? It's important to know the reasons you have to do this and justify it, so important people in your life will understand you, too.

To be able to do this, you should gather all the information you can get your hands on. However, always verify your sources. It can help to search about the low-carb diet's history and people who have experienced going through it. It can also help to know people who are using the diet as part of their lifestyle. Their contribution to your research can become valuable today and in the long run.

You can also use similar low-carb diets such as the Atkins Diet, which is popular today, as a reference. It's a diet used by many, including celebrities, to keep in tip-top shape.

Consult With Your Doctor

Knowing how successful many people are in their low-carb diets can make anyone dive into the craze without questions asked. This is dangerous and unhealthy, especially with people who have health issues. The only remedy is to consult your doctor before starting on this diet.

Limiting carb intake affects all people differently. What happens to one person may not happen to another person. What one experiences, may not be experienced by another. Doctors can best explain what happens to your body, so it's important to talk to them first. They can recommend steps that you can take, so you can safely undergo the low-carb diet without worrying about your health.

What's more, you will be experiencing some physical symptoms during your first few weeks under the low carb diet. Doctors can further explain what happens to the human body during this period.

Rally Support from Your Family and Friends (and Colleagues if necessary)

And here's why you should gather valid resources about the low-carb diet and why you should talk to your doctor first. Once you've informed your family and friends about what you're about to go through, many of them for sure will ask if you know what you're doing. Now, you can answer them properly and confidently.

After convincing them that you know what you're up against, tell them how rewarding this would be in the end – not only physically, but also health-wise. It is a major positive change in your life. This way, you can have their support, which is crucial in the overall process of the low-carb diet. You will need all the support you can get, so you won't have to explain all the time why you're eating the way you do.

One of the most dreaded scenarios in the life of low-carb dieters are social events or family gatherings. If you were not able to inform your family and friends before starting on this diet, you may end up explaining yourself each time you attend one of those get-togethers. If you did your assignment, they may likely be considerate enough of your situation and may be able to prepare a few dishes just for you.

Now, one question remains:

SHOULD YOU START A LOW CARB DIET?

The decision to go start and adapt an eating lifestyle that's low in carb intake is huge. Most of the time, it is applied as a diet to lose extra weight. Whatever your fitness goal is, you should be prepared.

WHAT HAPPENS IN A LOW CARB DIET?

The general idea of the low-carb diet is to substitute foods that are bad sources of carbohydrates, or bad carbs, with good sources of carbohydrates, or good carbs.

While doing so, you'll have to learn how to restrict your intake of good carbs in the long run. You'll learn to focus on making carb choices that are healthier. Moreover, you'll learn to limit your sugar intake,

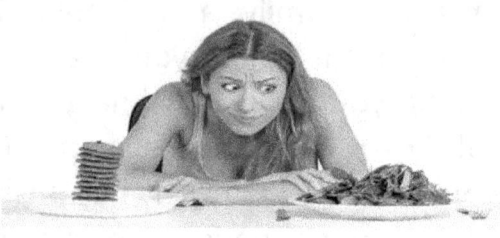

which can help you maintain a stable and healthy blood sugar level.

The Basic Science

The low-carb diet is all about taking out all the refined sugars and starches from your diet. There's no need to buy specially-made products, or extra stuff. You just need to remove all sources of unhealthy starches and sugars, and limit your carb intake to a certain amount per day.

This does not mean that you will have to starve yourself. The remaining part of your diet will be taken from non-starchy vegetables, protein, and healthy fats, which are all sources of good carbs. While refined carbs and sugars will make your blood sugar rise and plummet aggressively, good carbs will make your blood sugar stable. Bad carbs can also make you crave for more of it. Good carbs, on the other hand, satisfy your hunger for longer periods of time, so you eat less.

The State of Ketosis

Soon, you'll notice that your body is changing. As you remove carbs from your diet, you'll enter a state of ketosis. In this state, your body's metabolism will be reset. Instead of burning sugar (or glucose) as energy fuel, your body will burn fats. From this stage onwards, you can eat foods high in fats, but you will still continue losing weight.

When there's an absence of sugar in the blood, the body uses stored fat to fuel energy for the muscles. This is the secret of the low-carb diet and everybody loves it. You can eat "fattening" foods, but are still able to shed weight fast.

Ketosis Symptoms

While you're in a ketosis state, you'll experience heightened mood and bursts of energy, which are two major benefits of ketosis. Others include:

- Lowers insulin levels
- Increases your body's fat-burning ability
- You burn more calories
- Keeps appetite in control
- Promotes muscle growth
- Reduces excess water in the body

On the other hand, ketosis symptoms can cause keto-flu. It is a group of flu-like symptoms that include headache and nausea. Don't worry though, your body is just adapting to the changes you're making. Make sure to drink lots of water, including salted meat broth during this period.

Milder symptoms such as change in breath odor can signal that your body has already reached the ketosis state. Just to make sure, you can use keto strips to test your urine if it has ketones in it – a clear indication of ketosis state.

Finally:

STARTING ON THE LOW CARB DIET

The typical low-carb diet includes four phases. You start with the induction phase which is the most restrictive part of the diet. It lasts for 2 weeks.

Phase 1: The Induction Phase. In this phase, you can only eat a maximum of 40 grams of carbohydrates per day for the next 14 days. The rest of your diet comes from fat, protein, and leafy green vegetables.

Phase 2: The Balancing Phase. In this phase, you can gradually add small amounts of nuts, fruits, and low-carb vegetables. You'll start to notice a little weight loss here.

Phase 3: The Fine-Tuning Phase. In this phase, you have already lost a considerable amount of weight, though you haven't reached your weight goal yet. You can add more low-carb foods in your diet until weight loss slows down.

Phase 4: The Maintenance Phase. In this phase, you have already reached your weight goal. In order to maintain it, you have to eat healthy carbs only. You also eat healthy sources of protein and fats.

However, these phases are not all necessary. As long as you keep away from bad carbs, you can lose weight and maintain it for good.

WHAT ELSE YOU NEED TO KNOW

Learn to Count Carbs

The success of your low-carb diet depends on how many carbs you eat per day. You can only know this if you learn how to count carbs. In order to do this, you should develop the habit of reading food labels. Here's how in four easy steps:

1. Look at the food label and know the serving size. For example, serving size of a peanut butter is 2 tablespoons or 32 grams.
2. Get the total carbohydrates. For example, in this case let's use 7 grams.
3. Get the dietary fiber. For example, 2 grams.
4. Take out 2 grams from 7 grams and that is equal to 5 grams. That means that for every 2 tablespoon of peanut butter, you get 5 net carbs.

In other words, counting carbs is simply: total carbohydrates − dietary fiber = net carbs. Now, the tricky part is counting unpacked whole foods. Once you've learned how to count net carbs of packed foods, you can use this as a basis for net carbs of whole foods. To be sure, you can use the USDA National Nutrient Database to correctly determine the carb content of foods without packaging.

Carb-Proof Your Kitchen

Nothing will make your efforts harder than the presence of bad carbs in your kitchen. Before you start the low-carb diet, you need to remove all candy bars, cookies, potato chips, pasta, white bread, ice cream, and white rice from your kitchen.

Low-Carb Diet Shopping

Shopping for food while on a low-carb diet is different compared to a normal diet. You only have to buy low-carb foods and good sources of carbohydrates. To do this, you must learn how to create your own list of low carb foods and good carbs. In time, you'll learn to avoid grocery aisles that have high-carbs in them. In a separate chapter, you'll learn more about this.

Monitor Your Progress

From start to finish, you should keep track of your moves. Each step should be taken down on a fitness diary including your body weight, measurements, and body fat percentage. This can help you monitor your progress, especially your improvements. Taking before and after photos is also a big motivational tool. You'll see the amazing changes.

PREPARING LOW CARB MEALS

Every start of the week, you should create your own meal plan. A structured meal plan can help you avoid unnecessary food intake that can lead to a binge. It can also help lessen the stress of having to think about what to eat next. A well-planned meal ensures that you are able to eat the right amount of carbs in order to keep up with your new diet.

Lastly, you should know something about:

TIME AND COMMITMENT

The low-carb diet takes time for anyone to adjust to. It also involves commitment because meal planning is not an easy task. You need to make your diet enjoyable, while challenging. It's all worth it when you'll see the results. Focus on that.

Chapter 2: Getting Started

You can't just dismiss the benefits of the low carb diet. Aside from quick and easy weight loss, your health will experience a whole lot of improvement. You'll start to feel more energetic. You'll sleep better, feel stronger, and look younger. Your body can now have a strong resistance against diseases, and you'll lessen chances of inflammation in your body.

These promises are real, but only after you and your body have learned to adjust. All it takes is two weeks.

TWO WEEKS ON LOW CARB

Getting started with the low carb diet involves a two-week critical part. As mentioned in the first chapter, you are only allowed 40 grams of carbohydrates per day for the next two weeks, making this phase the most restrictive one. It's also dramatic.

Being introduced to a new eating lifestyle can psychologically, physically, and emotionally derail anyone. This is the work of your body's metabolism. Various bodily hormones are at work as your metabolism is being rewired for a new process.

However, there's a way to make this work for you. Considering the maximum carb intake per day is at 40 grams, you can change it a bit every single day as long as you keep the maximum requirement. For example, on a 3-day period, you can alternate between 40g – 30g – 40g. This method can make it easier for you to start. You can lessen the amount as you progress.

The Atkins Diet requires its dieters to eat 20 grams of carbs per day for two weeks. Now that's a bit harsh, but if you can start on that path, you can always do so. Here are some start-up tips:

- Don't forget to keep track of your carb intake for the first two weeks. Include this in your fitness diary.

- Drink lots of water, including salted broth.

- While you should always count your

carbs, counting your calories is not required for this diet.

- Never starve yourself. Always eat plenty of food, but avoid unhealthy sources of carbs, protein, and fats – which leads us to what you should and should not eat while on a low-carb diet.

Your New Plate

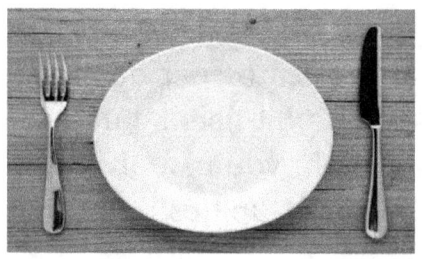

It's easier to create low-carb meal plans when you know which foods to avoid. For the first two weeks, you should not be eating the following:
Foods You Should Avoid

- any fruits

- milk
- nuts
- rice
- pasta
- bread
- alcoholic drinks
- artificially sweetened drinks
- chips
- candies
- ice cream
- chocolates
- deli meats
- highly processed foods
- packed, shredded cheese
- potatoes and other starchy vegetables
- oysters
- pork liver

Even low-carb alternatives of these foods are not allowed. Being a low-carb dieter means you should be adept at reading food labels. Reading them can help you determine if what you're eating has any of the foods mentioned above, especially milk and nuts.

During the two-week period, you'll also learn if you are allergic or sensitive to certain food types such as gluten. This way, you can easily avoid such foods in the future.

Foods You Can Eat

Without any of the foods above, your new plate for 2 weeks should include the following:

Meat, Poultry, and Fish

Majority of meats, fish, and poultry are zero in carbs. Always go for the fresh, unprocessed varieties.

Vegetables

Most vegetables have carbohydrates in them, but they are the healthier option. They don't make your blood sugar levels rise, or your unhealthy cravings start-up. In fact, they make you feel full longer, and keep your blood sugar levels stable. For the most part of your low-carb diet, you'll be sourcing your carbs from veggies. This does not include potatoes and starchy vegetables.

Eggs, Cheese, and Other Dairy Products

Eggs only have less than 1 gram of carbohydrates, so they're allowed. Heavy cream, cream cheese, cottage cheese, hard cheeses (Parmesan and Cheddar), and full-fat cheeses are also allowed.

Oils and Butter

Always choose healthy oils such as olive oil, fish oil (rich in Omega-3 fatty acids, which is good for the heart), and avocado oil. Coconut oil is also a healthy oil, but we'll discuss that separately. Butter is also a healthy oil, not the margarine variety. However, you should make sure that your butter was made using organic milk. Grass-fed cows produce healthier milk compared to cows fed with grains.

Coconut Oil

Coconut oil is one of the best choices of healthy oils. Not only is it an excellent source of healthy fat, it also helps your body burn more fat while you're in keto state. It boosts metabolism and lessens your unhealthy cravings. It tastes and smells great, too. However, make sure that you'll use virgin coconut oil only.

Herbs

Like vegetables, herbs also have small amounts of carbs in them. They can be used liberally considering they are a healthier option and the carbs in them are too little to count.

MEAL PORTIONS

To get the best results during your first two weeks, you should divide your macros (fats, protein, and carbs) using a respective ratio of 65%, 30%, and 5%.

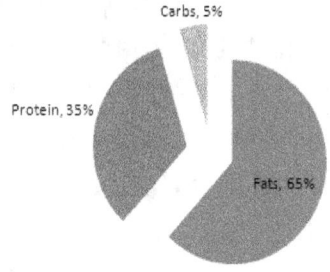

However, you can always modify this according to your body needs. For example, if you're aiming for a more tolerable start, which is 10-40 grams per day, your daily diet should look like any of these:

To discover the right levels of macros for your body, increase your carb intake and lessen your fats by small amounts. Track your progress for every adjustment you'll make, so you can see which combination is right for you.

A DAY TO DAY LOOK AT THE FIRST TWO WEEKS

Days 1-2: First 2 Days

The first two days is as important as the first two weeks of the low carb diet. Here, you'll start to break your body's craving for more carbs and sugar. As a result, the first 2 days are extra challenging. Your body has been used to burning glucose and carbs to fuel muscles and bodily functions. Now, you're teaching your body to use fats instead.

For the first 2 days, you'll feel cranky, shaky, and tired. You'll crave for sugary, high-carb foods. If you'll experience worse symptoms other than these, that means your body is addicted to sugar more than you first imagined.

Another reason why these 2 days are important is because glucose levels in your body can last for only 2 to 3 days. By avoiding carbs during these days, you're preventing your body from storing more glucose as its source of energy. It will only burn what's left in your body's stored glucose.

A recommended day to start your low-carb diet is on Friday night. This way, you can spend your first two days at the comfort of your own home. You can be cranky all day without having to put up with people from work or school. By the third day on Monday, you'll be moving on to the next part of the diet's first phase.

Days 3-7: Changing Metabolism

On the third day, because you have depleted your body's storage of glucose, it will start to burn fats and protein as its source of energy. Having a steady source of energy, your body will start to work normally again. Your brain starts to clear-up and you'll feel lively and energetic once again.

You should be increasing your intake of fats while you reduce your carb intake more. If your body has more stored healthy fats, you'll have more fuel to burn for your energy. Don't worry about overeating healthy fats because it's not necessarily easy to overeat them. You're not planning on drinking healthy oils, are you?

At this rate, your metabolism is now different. You no longer burn sugar and carbs, but only fats and protein.

Day 8-14: Rapid Weight Loss

After a week, you'll start to feel better. You'll have more energy and you'll be less cranky. Your roller coaster sugar levels will be gone. You will not feel shaky anymore when you're hungry. Your mood swings are now less. What's best, you might experience a little drop in your weight during this period.

You can now finally, and gradually, reintroduce carbs into your diet. You can now include low-carb foods in your meals, while maintaining your fat and protein intake.

AFTER THE FIRST TWO WEEKS

During this period, you should now be able to:

- Know how to count carbs
- Know what foods to avoid
- Know what foods are nutritious and are allowed to eat
- Maintain drinking 8 glasses or more of water ever day
- Remove all traces of high carb, sugary, junk foods from the kitchen

On the third week, it's time to review your progress. Make sure you have monitored your diet for the past two weeks. If you've lost weight, then that's good. Stay on Phase 1 until you've reached your weight goal. If nothing has changed, consider changing your strategy by adjusting your macros. Don't forget to keep track of your adjustments, so you know which one is working for you.

MAINTENANCE: ADD MORE CARBS INTO YOUR DIET

When you've already reached your weight goal, you can add more carbs into your diet. Eat good carbs only to avoid your sugar levels plummeting and rising back again. For each week, you can add 5 grams of good carbs into your diet. You'll notice that you're not losing weight anymore, but you're not gaining it either.

To help guide you in buying the right foods and which ones to add to your diet, let's move on to the next chapter.

Chapter 3: Low Carb Style Food Shopping

While you already know which foods to avoid and eat during the first two weeks of your low-carb diet, you still don't know which ones to include until you are able to maintain your weight. It's a bit tricky, especially when you're doing your best to avoid aisles in the grocery stores that have "forbidden" food items in them. Here's a 3-step strategy that can help you shop for your low-carb foods.

3-Step Strategy Plan for Buying Low Carb Foods

Step 1: Prepare Your Grocery List

Before you go to the grocery store, you should prepare your own grocery list. This can save you time and money. You know what needs to be bought, so you know where to go straight to once you're in the shop. It saves you money because a grocery list helps you avoid buying items that you don't really need. Here's another money-saving tip: stock up on vegetables. They're the most inexpensive, yet healthiest foods in your grocery list.

Considering you're still not familiar with maintaining your weight while on a low-carb diet, you can use the food list from your first two weeks as a guide.

Step 2: Stick to the Perimeter

Once you're in the grocery store, avoid visiting the inner aisles as much as possible. They contain majority of high carb, processed foods. The best way to do this is to shop around the edges of the grocery store. It is where most of the whole, fresh foods are located – a place where almost all foods are low-carb.

You can start at the vegetable and fruits section, then move on to the deli or meat section, don't forget the fish, and then to the dairy and eggs. If you need to buy other things, go only to the aisles that you need to. Don't go to sections that are not included in your grocery list. Just look at them, but don't go visit the aisles.

Step 3: Buy at the Local Farmer's Market or Butcher Store

If there are items in your grocery list that are not in the grocery store, you can always buy at the local farmer's market.

Even big cities have one. Visiting farmers are always eager to show their cream of the crop. You're getting organic, healthy foods at their best. Their produce is also inexpensive because they don't have to go through the process of repacking. Pre-cut, packaged veggies and fruits from grocery stores are pricier because of the lengthy process they go through.

Aside from supporting local farmers, you can buy cheaper alternatives of your meat choices from a local butcher.

These techniques sound easy. If you focus on your end goal, you know that what you're doing will be worth it. Now is not the time to act based on your instincts. Be always prepared when going to the grocery store.

WHAT SHOULD BE INCLUDED IN YOUR GROCERY LIST

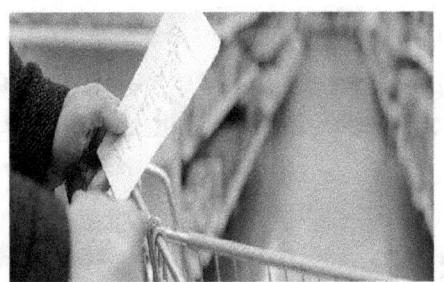

After your first two weeks, you can include the following in your grocery list:

Meat, Fish and Seafood, Poultry and Eggs

Meat is a staple in the low carb diet. You should always include these in your cart. If you're still in the induction phase, avoid pork liver and oysters. They have carbs in them. Eggs are low in carbs and a good source of healthy fat.

Here's a more specific list:

Meats and Poultry	*Deli Meats*	*Fish and Seafood*
• Ground beef • Beef tips and steaks • Pork and	• Prosciutto • Bologna and salami • Pepperoni slices or sticks • Cold cuts such	• Fresh or frozen fish • Fresh or canned salmon

beef roasts • Pork and beef ribs • Pork chops, loins, and steaks • Sausage, ham, and bacon • Chicken (whole or parts) • Ground turkey	as pastrami (but check for added sugars) and turkey breast	• Tuna in oil or water • Fresh or frozen shrimps • Fresh or frozen scallops • Crab • Lobster • Oysters and mussels

Dairy and Cheese

You can now add this to your diet: full-fat yoghurt, Greek yoghurt (plain or full-fat only), ricotta, soft cheeses (Farmer's and Muenster), and sour cream.

Healthy Oils and Fat

Avoid hydrogenated oils, even partially-hydrogenated ones. They are not good for your health. Stick to oils high in Omega-3 fatty acids, such as fish oil. They're good for the heart.

Frozen Food

While processed foods are not allowed in the induction phase, you can now eat frozen foods. Just don't forget to read the labels. Check out how many carbs and dietary fiber are included in them.

Frozen foods are also perfect for meal preparations. They make everything quick, so you save time and energy. Alternatively, you can buy your fresh groceries, cut them up, divide them into bags and freeze them. You can do this with your meats, fish, and poultry as well.

Canned Goods

Like with frozen foods, you have to read labels when you're buying canned goods. They are also a great way to save time and energy.

However, avoid canned fruits with heavy syrup or canned veggies that have high sodium content. Go for canned soy or black beans, olives, and unsweetened coconut milk. Here's a full list of allowed canned goods for the low carb diet:

Nut Butters	Choose natural and unsweetened. Don't forget to refrigerate them after opening.
Stock	Chicken and vegetable stock
Canned Veggies	Sauerkraut Green chilies, chipotle peppers, and roasted red peppers Mushrooms Artichoke hearts Green beans Hearts of palm Okra (check labels for added sugar though)
Sauces	Pasta sauce including Alfredo sauce with no thickener or added sugar Pizza sauce
Tomato Products	Tomato paste, tomato sauce, sun-dried tomatoes in oil (even adding a little gives a lot of flavor), and canned tomatoes. Always look for brands with the lowest net carb content.
Meat	Aside from the ones mentioned

under the meat section above, you can add sardines and anchovies, Vienna sausages and canned luncheon meat, but only in small portions. Real meat is still healthier.

Nuts and Seeds

Products made from nuts and seeds are always healthy choices. Flour, milk, butter, and oils made from almond, flaxseed, and coconut are always the best. They are also perfect for baking purposes. Others include:

Nuts	*Seeds*
• Almonds • Hazelnuts • Macadamia nuts • Walnuts • Pecans	• Sesame seeds • Pumpkin seeds • Sunflower seeds

You can create your own trail mix using these nuts. Freeze them to make them last longer.

Condiments and Spices

Some spices actually boost your body's weight loss ability, especially while you're in keto. To increase your body's fat-burning power, add the following in your diet:

- Mustard
- High-fat salad dressing
- Soy sauce (unless you're sensitive to gluten)
- Hot sauce
- Pesto sauce
- Full-fat mayonnaise
- Dill pickle relish
- Bouillon/broth cubes
- Salsa
- Vinegar: Wine vinegar and apple cider vinegar. Use balsamic vinegar in small amounts only
- Capers, olives, and horseradish
- Lemon or lime juice

When choosing your condiments, always be on the lookout for unsweetened, sugar-free or no-added sugar ones. You should go for these kinds. Avoid ones with sugar.

Artificial Sweeteners

Sucralose (like Splenda) and saccharine (like Sweet N' Low) can be included in your food list. However, they should be taken in small amounts only. All natural alternatives such as Erythritol and Stevia are also allowed.

Cooking and Baking Ingredients

If you know how to bake, you can always make your own low-carb dessert alternatives. Here's what you can use on the low-carb diet:

- Flour: good alternatives are made from almond, coconut and other nuts. Always store your low-carb flour in the freezer to make them last longer past their expiration dates.
- For binding and thickening, you can use xantham gum
- Flavoring and coloring extracts such as almond, lemon, and vanilla. Check for

added sugar, which you must avoid.
- Include whey protein powder, which is good for shakes and meal replacement drinks. You can choose from chocolate, vanilla, and plain flavors.
- Unsweetened cocoa powder, or dark chocolate
- Plain, unsweetened gelatin
- Beef sticks or jerky
- Pork rinds. When crushed, they make a good substitute for bread crumbs.

Fruits and Vegetables

Fruits and vegetables are always good sources of good carbs. While fruits are not allowed in the induction phase, you can now eat them (but sparingly). When you've reached your target weight, fruits can be added as much as you want.

Leafy green and brightly-colored vegetables are still in. You're still now allowed to eat starchy vegetables however.

Fruits and veggies are last in the list because the full detailed-list is quite long. Here are the most recommended ones:

Low-Carb Fruits (serving, net carbs in grams)

- Acai Berry, 1 oz, 5g
- Apple, ½ piece, 8.7g
- Apricot, ¼ cup, 3g
- Avocado, ½ cup, 1g
- Banana, ½ of small, 10.1g
- Blackberries, ¼ cup, 2.7g
- Black Raspberries, ½ cup, 3.7g
- Blueberries, ¼ cup, 4g
- Cantaloupe, ½ cup, 7g
- Cherries, ¼ cup, 4.2g
- Coconuts, ¼ cup, 1.3g
- Cranberries, ¼ cup, 2g
- Kiwi, 1 whole, 8.7g
- Mango, ¼ cup, 6.3g
- Passion Fruit, ¼ cup, 7.7g
- Peach, 1 small, 7.2g
- Pears, ½ of medium, 10.3g
- Persimmon, ½ of small, 4.1g
- Pineapple, ¼ cup, 4.8g
- Plum, ¼ cup, 7.6g
- Pomegranate, ¼ of whole, 10g
- Prickly Pear, 1 whole, 6.2g
- Raisins, Golden, 1 tbsp, 6.8g
- Raisins, Seedless, 1 tbsp, 6.8g

- Currant, ¼ cup, 4g
- Elderberries, ¼ cup, 4g
- Gooseberries, ¼ cup, 9g
- Grapes, ¼ cup, 6.7g
- Grapefruit (red), ½ of whole, 7.9g
- Guava, ½ cup, 5.3g
- Honeydew, ¼ cup, 3.6g
- Lemon, ¼ cup, 3.5g
- Raspberries, ¼ cup, 1.7g
- Red Raspberries, ½ cup, 3.4g
- Rhubarb, ½ cup, 1.7g
- Starfruit, ¼ cup, 3g
- Strawberries, sliced, ½ cup, 4.7g
- Tangerine, 1 small, 8.8g
- Watermelon, ½ cup, 5.2g

Low-Carb Vegetables (serving, net carbs in grams)

- Alfalfa Sprouts, 1 cup/raw, 0.4g
- Argula, ½ cup/raw, 0.2g
- Artichoke Hearts, 1/in water, 1.0g
- Leeks, ¼ cup/boiled, 1.7g
- Lettuce Iceberg, ½ cup, 0.1g
- Mushrooms ½ cup, 1.2g

- Asparagus, 6 stalks/boiled, 2.4g
- Avocado, 1 whole/raw, 3.5g
- Bamboo Shoots, 1 cup/boiled, 1.1g
- Beets, ½ cup/canned, 4.7g
- Bok Choy, 1, 0.8g
- Broccoli, ½ cup/boiled, 1.6g
- Brussels Sprouts, ¼ cup, 2.4g boiled
- Cabbage, ½ cup, 2.0g
- Cauliflower, ½ cup, 1.0g
- Celery, 1 stalk, 0.8g
- Chard, ½ cup Swiss, 1.8g boiled
- Chicory Greens, ½ cup/raw, 0.6g
- Chives, 1 tbs, 0.1g
- Collard Greens, ½ cup, 4.2g boiled
- Okra, ½ cup, 2.4g
- Olives, green, 5, 2.5g
- Olives, black, 5, 0.7g
- Onion, ¼ cup/raw, 2.8g
- Parsley, 1 tbs, 0.1g
- Peas, ½ cup podded, 3.4g
- Peppers, ½ cup/raw, 2.3g
- Pumpkin, ¼, cup/boiled, 2.4g
- Radicchio, ½ cup/raw, 0.7g
- Radishes, 10/raw, 0.9g
- Rhubarb, ½ cup, unsweetened, 1.7g
- Romaine Lettuce, ½ cup, 0.2g
- Sauerkraut, ½ cup canned, 1.2g
- Spaghetti Squash, ½ cup, 2.0g boiled

- Cucumber, ½ cup, 1.0g
- Daikon, ½ cup, 1.0g
- Eggplant, ½ cup, 1.8g
- Endive, ½ cup, 0.0g
- Escarole, ½ cup, 0.0g
- Fennel, 1 cup, 3.6g
- Jicama, ½ cup, 2.5g
- Kale, ½ cup, 2.4g
- Spinach, ½ cup, 0.2g raw
- Summer Squash, ½ cup, 2.0g boiled
- Tomato, 1 raw, 4.3g
- Turnips, ½ cup, 2.2g boiled
- Water Chestnuts, ½ cup/canned, 6.9g
- Zucchini, ½ cup sautéed, 2.0g

Now you know what to do, you should get started. Good luck!

Conclusion

"Time is free, but it's priceless. You can't own it, but you can use it. You can't keep it, but you can spend it. Once you've lost it you can never get it back.

Yes, it's sure and certain that time is like a river. As the current of the river flows ahead and never comes back. Same is with time. Once lost it can't be regained.

It's truly said that,"Don't count every hour in the day, make every hour in the day count."we got to be very punctual and studies in our lives about time.

The whole world runs along with it. If anyone remains back, he surely will be described as a loser in his life .It goes the same with famous Jim rohns as he says, Time is more valuable than money. You can get more money, but you cannot get more time.

Time is like money. Every day, hour, minute, second is precious for us. As we spend money wisely, in the same way our time should be spent very cautiously. For this time management is very essential.

Another famous maxim goes ,"A stitch in time saves nine". However we always misuse it. Its proper utilization is very necessary.

A farmer has to harvest his crops on time but if he neglects, the birds will eat those crops or untimely rain may destroy it.

A successful man only knows the value of time because he has come up with proper use of time joint with hard work. So, time should not be procrastinated instead every single second should be used carefully.

Then only a person will touch the sky of success.

About The Author

Cecil Jennings loves low carb cooking The author has written several recipe books on the topic. He has served as an instructor promoting various cusine arts in indie shows and fairs. He is currently living with his spouse in Texas.

www.ingramcontent.com/pod-product-compliance
Lightning Source LLC
LaVergne TN
LVHW020432080526
838202LV00055B/5151